Gislene Cordeiro da Silveira
Lilian A. da Silva

Physiotherapy for Alzheimer's patients

Gislene Cordeiro da Silveira
Lilian A. da Silva

Physiotherapy for Alzheimer's patients

Palliative Care for the Late-Stage Patient

ScienciaScripts

Imprint

Any brand names and product names mentioned in this book are subject to trademark, brand or patent protection and are trademarks or registered trademarks of their respective holders. The use of brand names, product names, common names, trade names, product descriptions etc. even without a particular marking in this work is in no way to be construed to mean that such names may be regarded as unrestricted in respect of trademark and brand protection legislation and could thus be used by anyone.

Cover image: www.ingimage.com

This book is a translation from the original published under ISBN 978-613-9-68287-4.

Publisher:
Sciencia Scripts
is a trademark of
Dodo Books Indian Ocean Ltd. and OmniScriptum S.R.L publishing group

120 High Road, East Finchley, London, N2 9ED, United Kingdom
Str. Armeneasca 28/1, office 1, Chisinau MD-2012, Republic of Moldova, Europe
Printed at: see last page
ISBN: 978-620-8-20627-7

SUMMARY

THANKS

I would first like to thank God for helping me on this journey, giving me the wisdom, understanding and strength to achieve my goals;

To my parents Ana Lucia and Willian for believing in my ability, being my foundations, supporting and encouraging me to make my dream come true;

To my aunt and uncle Carlos and Sandra, my grandmother Zélia, my sisters who were by my side believing in this achievement;

To my husband for encouraging me and being by my side;

To my friends for their companionship;

To the professors for their dedication and teaching;

To Professor Lilian Atalaia, for her guidance in the preparation of this work, collaborating in the development of my ideas and contributing to my learning;

"There can be no healing without care, but there can be care even without healing."

(MADELEINE LENINGER)

SUMMARY

INTRODUCTION: The elderly population is the fastest growing segment in the country. The aging of the population also reflects a change in various aspects, such as economic, social and health. In this context, neurodegenerative pathologies have gained importance in the current scenario, among them Alzheimer's disease. Alzheimer's is a neurodegenerative disease with a progressive decline in cognition and is divided into three stages: mild, moderate and severe. When the patient is in this last phase, special, humanized care is advisable, seeking to provide pain relief and quality of life within the limitations of the disease. Palliative care is an approach to promoting the quality of life of patients and their families facing diseases that cannot be cured, providing relief from suffering, comfort and preventing further complications. Physiotherapy is of the utmost importance in this care, with appropriate treatment for each patient, using resources, techniques and exercises.

OBJECTIVE: The aim of this study is to highlight the importance of palliative care, especially physiotherapy, for patients with a clinical diagnosis of severe Alzheimer's disease.

METHODOLOGY: This is a clinical case report, in which the patient investigated has a diagnosis of Alzheimer's and is in the severe phase. A physiotherapeutic assessment was carried out in order to analyze muscle trophism, the patient's general history, medications used, time since diagnosis of the pathology, as well as the period he is bedridden. The treatment plan was based on the Palliative Care Manual.

RESULT: Although the patient's condition continued, pain relief was observed during the treatment, as the patient's face appeared more serene to the therapeutic touch, without expressing behaviors that indicated discomfort or pain. Physiotherapy is therefore an important palliative care tool for patients with advanced Alzheimer's disease.

Keywords: Palliative care. Physiotherapy Alzheimer's disease

1 INTRODUCTION

1.1 SOCIO-DEMOGRAPHIC AGEING

According to the Statute of the Elderly, a person is considered elderly when they reach the age of 60 (LEI 10741; DE 01.10.2003, ART.1). According to data from the Brazilian Institute of Geography and Statistics (IBGE), the elderly population is the fastest growing segment in the country. Between 2005 and 2015, the percentage of elderly people rose from 9.8% to 14.3%. At the same time as this growth, the portions of the population between 0 and 14 years old (known as children) and between 15 and 29 years old (young people) fell significantly. There is therefore a clear trend towards demographic ageing in Brazil.

Brazil has not prepared itself for the ageing of its country, its population has grown rapidly, without planning to accommodate the elderly population, which is growing at a much faster rate than the young population. The ageing of the population also reflects a change in various aspects, such as economic, social and health. In terms of health, there has been a shift from infectious and parasitic diseases to chronic degenerative diseases, precisely because of the increase in life expectancy (MACHADO, 2006).

In this sense, many neurodegenerative pathologies have acquired importance in the current scenario, among which Alzheimer's disease stands out.

1.2 ALZHEIMER

Alzheimer's disease is a neurodegenerative disease with a progressive decline in cognition (COELHO, 2010). The neuropathology is characterized by two mechanisms: the formation of amyloid plaques outside the neurons and the formation of neurofibrillary tangles inside the neurons. These mechanisms lead to brain atrophy, especially in areas such as the hippocampus and the entorhinal cortex, which are responsible for processing recent memory, and also atrophy of the basal nucleus of Meynert together with the septal nuclei in the medial forebrain, which are responsible for producing the neurotransmitter acetylcholine, which is important for cognitive processing. As the disease progresses, the entire cerebral cortex becomes affected, and consequently other cognitive functions are compromised, including behavioral disorders.

According to the Brazilian Alzheimer's Association (ABRAZ, 2012), the disease is divided into three phases: mild, moderate and severe. The mild or initial phase is where minor forgetfulness, depressive symptoms and loss of a sense of time and space begin. In the moderate phase, the patient is no longer able to carry out their daily activities, has difficulty forming sentences, has a sudden change in behavior, can even become aggressive, needs help with personal hygiene and can't remember the names of people close to them. And finally, in the advanced stage, which will be addressed in this study, the patient is already debilitated, with total dependence on their basic activities of daily living, has clinical complications, notable difficulty communicating, no recognition of family and self, presence of primitive reflexes (such as fetal position). When the patient is in this last phase, special, humanized care is advisable, seeking to provide pain relief and quality of life within the limitations of the disease.

1.3 PALLIATIVE CARE AND PHYSIOTHERAPY

In 2002, the World Health Organization (WHO) defined palliative care as an approach to promote the quality of life of patients and their families, who face diseases that have no diagnosis of cure, correct evaluation and humanized treatment through prevention, relief of suffering, pain and unpleasant symptoms, always respecting the patient's limits. When a progressive and incurable disease affects a family environment, it causes a great deal of inconvenience for the patient and their family. Because of this, palliative care uses a multi-professional team made up of a doctor, psychologist, physiotherapist and social worker, who treats the patient and family in a humanized way, taking care of their physical, psychological, social and spiritual needs. At this stage of the disease, the caregiver/family is not prepared to deal with such a situation, due to emotional reasons, lack of information and/or financial problems.

The professionals in the multidisciplinary team are all important in palliative care. However, this work aims to show how important physiotherapy is in this care, with appropriate treatment for each patient, using resources, techniques and exercises, providing pain relief, and offering support for both the patient and their family.

According to MARCCUC (2005) physiotherapy has a large number of useful intervention methods in palliative care. And this treatment is not just physical, it is aimed at the individual as a whole, so physiotherapy in palliative care is very important for the patient's comfort and also to give them more dignity while coping with the disease.

According to BRAGA; ROSA; NOGUEIRA (2008), physiotherapists play a significant role in health promotion and disease prevention through information and guidance for activities of daily living (ADLs), prevention of deformities, postural care, care for sequelae after musculoskeletal, neuromuscular and cardiopulmonary alterations when the disease is already installed and social reintegration, knowing the context in which the individual being assisted lives.

This research aims to show the relevance of physiotherapeutic conduct with palliative care for patients at an advanced stage of Alzheimer's disease, it is at this stage that they are debilitated with total dependence on their activities, Physiotherapy contemplates several aspects such as neurological, respiratory and cardiac to give the patient a humanized and quality treatment, providing analgesia and reducing discomfort due to being bedridden.

In addition to playing an important role in the treatment, such as preventing joint deformities, shortening and trophism, generated by immobility, it also provides help and guidance to carers and their families at this difficult time.

1.4 MUSICOTHERAPY

Allied to physiotherapy treatment, music therapy has proved to be an important complementary tool. According to ALBURQUEQUE (2012) music has the effect of evoking feelings of happiness and nostalgia, non-verbal communication, pain reduction, ease of body movements in the elderly, well-being, relaxation and comfort. According to Cunha (1999), even as the disease progresses, music therapy manages to communicate, stimulate memory, and reorganize the cognitive, affective and bodily functions of those suffering from the disease.

The use of music therapy in Alzheimer's patients is considerably satisfactory, as it increases the level of well-being, reducing depressive symptoms, stress and anxiety (ORTi, 2014).

2. GENERAL OBJECTIVE

The aim of this study is to highlight the importance of palliative care, especially physiotherapy, for patients with a clinical diagnosis of severe Alzheimer's disease.

2.1 SPECIFIC OBJECTIVES

- Maintaining the range of movement of the main joints

- Promoting comfortable postures

- Promote proper breathing rhythm

- Maintaining the correct functioning of physiological functions

- Providing bronchial hygiene

- Treating and preventing complications such as pressure ulcers and limb edema

3. METHODOLOGY

This is a home-based clinical case report. The patient under investigation has a clinical diagnosis of Alzheimer's, is in the severe stage, and has been bedridden for 2 years due to 2 episodes of cerebral ischemia.

First of all, an analysis was made of the patient's general history, time since diagnosis of the pathology, medication used, period of being bedridden, promoting a clinical study of the patient, a physiotherapeutic assessment was carried out with the patient in dorsal decubitus, in order to analyze the measurement of passive range of motion (ROM) (using the goniometer) in the upper limb joints glenohumeral, acromioclavicular, scapulohumeral, ulnar, radial humeral and carpometacarpal joints, and the lower limb hip, knee and ankle joints, to assess muscle shortening, and to analyze breathing patterns through observation and lung auscultation. It should be noted that information on the anamnesis, except for the physical examination, was collected from the patient's caregiver, since the patient is no longer able to understand and respond coherently. The caregiver also signed a consent form for the research to be carried out.

The treatment plan was based on the Palliative Care Manual (2013), created by the World Health Organization (WHO), comprising the following aspects:

- Acquiring a comfortable posture that favors breathing

- Mobilization and stretching of respiratory muscles for ventilatory improvement

- Breathing exercises for inhalation and exhalation, with the patient blowing into a straw with a glass of water, with the aim of increasing airflow to dislodge mucus, and strengthening the respiratory muscles by performing them 3 times for 10 seconds each. Lip crimping to improve ventilation and oxygenation, performed 3 times lasting 10 seconds each,

- Positioning and changes of position every 2 hours (transfers from bed to wheelchair/armchair/bath chair - guidance for caregivers)

- Passive stretching of the muscles of the upper limbs and lower limbs to prevent contracture and maintain ROM

- Joint mobilization to restore arthrokinematic movement, preventing immobility and its consequences such as deformity,

- Relaxing massage therapy using gliding and kneading on the upper limbs

and lower limbs;

It is worth mentioning that music therapy was used throughout the treatment

as a complementary form of treatment, since it provides a relaxing and

comfortable sensation, giving a humanized and quality treatment.

4. RESULTS

This is a clinical case study of an 81-year-old male patient who has been clinically diagnosed with late-onset or advanced Alzheimer's disease for over 8 years (medical report is attached). He has been confined to bed for 2 years due to 2 episodes of cerebral ischemia, and has little verbal comprehension and expression.

The drugs used by the patient are Donopezila to prevent the disease from progressing, Sinvastatin for cholesterol, Ass to thin the blood, Karvil to speed up the heart and prevent fatigue, Finasteride and Doxazosin for the prostate, Citalopram, Tradazone and Quetiapine for calming.

According to the fundamentals of palliative care, the patient is treated by a multidisciplinary team: a neurologist, a speech therapist (the speech therapist's report is attached as Annex B) and a nutritionist. The physiotherapy part of this study was carried out by the researcher, who will focus on physiotherapeutic treatment.

Fifteen sessions were held, three times a week, every other day, lasting 60 minutes each. Before and after each session, blood pressure was measured, and lung auscultation was performed at the assessment and reassessment, detecting the presence of vesicular murmur, without adventitious noises

During the assessment, the presence of a pressure sore in the coccygeal region was noted (photo is attached as Annex C), where the patient was instructed to clean himself with warm water, saline and ointment and to change his position every 2 hours, positioning himself correctly and protecting his extremities (photo of positioning is attached as Annex D), the patient has deformity of the fingers (clawed fingers), tremor when moving quickly, stiffness in the glenohumeral, acromioclavicular, scapulohumeral, ulnar, radial humeral and carpometacarpal joints of the upper limbs, and in the hip, knee and ankle joints of the lower limbs.

With regard to muscles, there was a shortening of the upper muscles pectoralis major, upper trapezius, deltoid, biceps and triceps brachii, flexors and extensors, and in the lower limb the quadriceps femoris muscle, abductors, adductors, extensors, has urinary and fecal incontinence (uses a diaper), has no trunk control, does not walk.

The table below shows the degree of ADM before treatment:

ADM	PRE
ELBOW FLEXION D	50°
BENDING AND	40°
SHOULDER FLEXION D	80°
BENDING AND	60°
ABDUCTION ARM D	50°
WELCOME AND	80°
QUADRICEPS FLEXAO D	50°
BENDING AND	40°

It was observed during treatment that there was no change in ADM's with passive movements.

ADM	PRE	POST-INTERVENTION
ELBOW FLEXION D	50°	50°
BENDING AND	40°	40°
SHOULDER FLEXION D	80°	80°
FLEXION E	60°	60°
ABDUCTION ARM D	50°	50°
E-ABDUCTION	80°	80°
FLEXION QUADRICEPS D	50°	50°
FLEXION AND	40°	40°

The ulcer remained, but with less intensity, and the patient continued to have adequate pulmonary auscultation. Despite the persistence of the condition, it was observed that there was better tolerance to therapeutic touch during treatment, since the patient's face appeared more serene, without expressing

behaviors that indicated discomfort or pain. This behavior was enhanced

during music therapy.

5. DISCUSSION

The purpose of palliative care is to provide assistance at the end of life, when the patient has a progressive disease and there is no hope of a cure. This care prepares the individual for the so-called "good death" (FLORIANI , SCHRAMM, 2013), because it aims to provide the individual with comfort and prepare them for the end of life in a dignified way, without suffering, without pain and being able to be at home with their family members, often instead of in a more impersonal environment such as a hospital bed.

According to CRUZ (2014), the role of the physiotherapist in palliative care is important in preventing the resulting alterations such as immobilization, joint stiffness, preventing the functional and early loss that occurs in patients with dementia.

In the study by GIRÂO, ALVES (2013), it is concluded that physiotherapy in palliative care is a global approach, as the patient is in the terminal stage, and the objective contributes positively to the quality of life, pain relief and promotes well-being to the patient, optimizing functionality until death.

In the present study, the patient responded well to the music stimulus, although he was no longer able to express himself verbally, his face clearly became more serene when he was mobilized while listening to the ambient music. Despite being subjective and difficult to measure, the professional who cares for this type of patient, with a high level of complexity, must be aware of the subtleties that go beyond quantified acts.

The study by SEKI and GALHEIGO (2010) obtained the same result regarding music with patients beyond the possibility of a cure, providing the patient with comfort and quality of life.

The result of this study was a positive response to the patient's tolerance to touch during the exercises, but he maintained the same joint angles as at the start of treatment. To our knowledge, there have been no studies to date showing gains in patients with advanced Alzheimer's when using palliative care. Therefore, more interventional studies need to be carried out.

OLIVEIRA (2015) states the importance of the multidisciplinary team in the treatment of palliative care and emphasizes the importance of the physiotherapy professional through muscle stretching, pain relief and improvement in the execution of movements. These principles were upheld during this case study, since the patient can be looked at from different professional perspectives.

According to CAZEIRO, PERES (2010), bedridden patients have reduced diaphragmatic movement, reduced ventilation, difficulty in eliminating secretions, can have complications such as pneumonia and atelectasis and can generate an accumulation of fluid at the base of the lung.

In the study by SPOSITO and TELLINI (1993), correct positioning is aimed at preventing ulcers, selecting an appropriate mattress, pillows, foams and others to protect the joints.

Despite knowing about the course of the disease and its prognosis, physiotherapy treatment was able to stabilize symptoms and prevent problems such as accumulation of secretions, fixed deformities, pressure ulcers, among others. But more than preventing problems, physiotherapy was an important tool, integrated into palliative care, to promote analgesia, comfort and dignity until the moment, inherent to all, which is departure.

However, it was very difficult to find articles related to palliative care in patients

with Alzheimer's disease.

6. CONCLUSION

This study showed the importance of physiotherapy in palliative care for patients with advanced Alzheimer's disease.

Despite the maintenance of the patient's condition, it was very effective to observe a positive response to the patient's tolerance to touch during mobilization and the effect that music therapy offers, leaving the patient relaxed, helping to relieve the patient's pain and comfort.

7. BIBLIOGRAPHICAL REFERENCES.

ALBUQUERQUE, Maria Cicera S, NASCIMENTO, Luciana Oliveira do, LYRA, Sarah Taynà, TREZZA, Maria Cristina Soares Figueiredo, BRÊDA, Mércia Zeviani; Os efeitos da mùsica em idosos com doença de Alzheimer de uma instituição de longa permanência; **Rev. Eletr 2012** abr/jun;14(2):404-13.

Brazilian Alzheimer's Association (2012) Alzheimer's disease: the sooner you know, the longer you'll remember" available http://abraz.org.br/abraz-na HYPERLINK"http://abraz.org.br/abraz-na-

media/release-institutional-disease-of-alzheimer"media/release-institutional-disease-of-alzheimer.Date last accessed: February 2017

National Association for Palliative Care (2006). Organizing services in palliative care: ANCP recommendations. [Online]. Available: http://www.apcp.com.pt/uploads/RecomendacoesOrganizacaodeServicos.pdf Date last accessed: February 2017

BRAGA, A. F.; ROSA, K. O. L. C.; NOGUEIRA, R. L. Atuaçâo do fisioterapeuta nas equipes de saù da família. Investigaçâo. Sâo Paulo, v. 8 n. 1-3 p. 19-24, 2008

COELHO, Flâvia de Melo. Physical activity and frontal cognitive functions associated with kinematic gait parameters in patients with Alzheimer's dementia.

Rio Claro. July 2010.

CAZEIRO, Ana Paula, PERES, Patricia. Occupational Therapy in the Prevention and Treatment of Complications Resulting from Bed Immobilization. Cadernos de Terapia Ocupacional da UFSCar, Sâo Carlos, May/Aug. 2010, v. 18, n.2, p. 149-167

CUNHA, Rosemyriam. Music therapy for the elderly.

Tuiuti University of Paranà, 1999. Specialization monograph.

CRUZ, Helena Alexandra gomes, Clinical practice report, Role of physiotherapy in palliative care, November 2014.

ESTATUTO do idoso: lei federal n° 10.741, de 01 de outubro de 2003. Brasilia, DF:

Special Secretariat for Human Rights, 2004.

FLORIANI CA, Schramm FR. Palliative care: interfaces, conflicts and needs. **Cien Saude Colet** 2008;

GIRAO, Mariana; Alves, Sandra; Physiotherapy in palliative care, **esscup journal of health sciences;** vol 5; november 2013

IBGE-Brazilian Institute of Geography and Statistics,

Available at

http://www.ibge.gov.br/home/presidencia/noticias/25072002pidoso.shtm.

Date of last access 15 May 2017.

MACHADO, JCB. Alzheimer's disease. In: Freitas EV, Py L, **Tratado de Geriatria e Gerontologia** Guanabara Koogan, 2° ediçâo ,2006. Op. cit. p. 178-201

MARCUCCI, F. (2005). The role of the physiotherapist in palliative care for cancer patients. **Revista Brasileira de Cancerologia**. 51 (1), 6777

OLIVEIRA, Mariana Branco; The approach of patients with chronic pain and palliative care in the family health strategy. Rio de Janeiro 2015.

ORTI, José Enrique de la Rubia, ESPINÓS, Paula Sancho, IRANZO Carmen CABANÉS, Impacto fisiológico de la musicoterapia en la depresión, ansiedad, y bienestar del paciente con demencia tipo Alzheimer. Valoración de la utilización de cuestionarios para cuantificarlo, **Psychology and Education** 2014, Vol. 4, N° 2;

SEKI, N., H; GALHEIGO, S, M; The use of music in palliative care: humanizing care and making it easier to say goodbye ;2010

SPOSITO, M.M.M; TELLINI, G.G; ITAMI, R.K. Prophylaxis of complications resulting from prolonged restriction of the patient in bed. Acta Paulista de Enfermagem, v. 6, n. 1, p. 11-15, 1993.

APPENDIX A - INFORMED CONSENT FORM

INFORMED CONSENT FORM

You are being invited as a volunteer to take part in the research project "Physiotherapist involvement in palliative care for patients with advanced Alzheimer's disease". We believe that physiotherapists are needed at this stage of the disease to provide more humanized care with quality of life and appropriate treatment. Therefore, in this study we intend to evaluate muscle trophism, the patient's general history, medication used, time since the pathology was diagnosed, as well as the length of time the patient has been bedridden, promoting a clinical study of the patient, measuring active and passive range of motion (ROM) (using a goniometer), and analyzing respiratory patterns.

For this study, we will adopt the following procedures: a day will be set aside for an initial assessment, asking questions about the patient's general history, medication used, time since the pathology was diagnosed, as well as the length of time the patient has been bedridden, promoting a clinical study of the patient. For 15 days, cognitive stimulation, joint mobilization, stretching and relaxation will be offered three times a week, with each session lasting 60 minutes. All sessions will be supervised by the physiotherapist in charge. After 15 days, the volunteer will be assessed again (the same questions that were covered in the initial assessment).

As this is an exercise program, some risks, however small, may occur, such as fatigue and a rise in blood pressure. However, it should be emphasized that at all times the participant will be supervised by the physiotherapist and her duly trained health team, in order to avoid such risks and/or intervene when necessary. It is hoped that the program will only benefit the elderly in terms of actions that can prevent and reduce risks, as well as stimulating cognitive performance. If we find satisfactory effects from this program,

To take part in this study, you will not incur any costs or receive any financial benefits. You will be informed about the study in any way you wish and you are free to participate or refuse to participate. You may withdraw your consent or stop participating at any time. Your participation is voluntary and refusal to take part will not lead to any penalty or change in the way you are treated by the researchers.

The researchers will treat your identity with professional standards of confidentiality.

The results of the research will be made available to you when it is finished. Your name or any material indicating your participation will not be released without your permission.

You will not be identified in any publication that may result from this study.

This consent form is printed in two copies, one of which will be kept by the researcher in charge and the other will be given to you.

Me, ,

bearer of identity document ____

I have been informed of the objectives of the research study, "Physiotherapist

work with palliative care in patients with advanced Alzheimer's", in a clear and

detailed manner and have clarified my doubts. I know that at any time I can

request further information and change my decision to participate if I so wish.

I declare that I agree to take part in this study. I have received a copy of this

informed consent form and have been given the opportunity to read it and

clarify my doubts.

____
Signature of   participantDate

    Researcher's signatureDate

Signature of   witnessDate

If you have any questions about the ethical aspects of this study, you can

consult the Research Ethics Committee (CEP) - Rua Botucatu, 572 - 1° andar

- cj 14, 5571-1062,

FAX: 5539-7162 - E-mail: cepunifesp@unifesp.br

If you have any questions, please contact Lilian Atalaia da Silva directly: (32)

8843-7898; Rua Redentor 280, or via email: lilian.atalaia@gmail.com.

ANNEX: A NEUROLOGIST'S REPORT

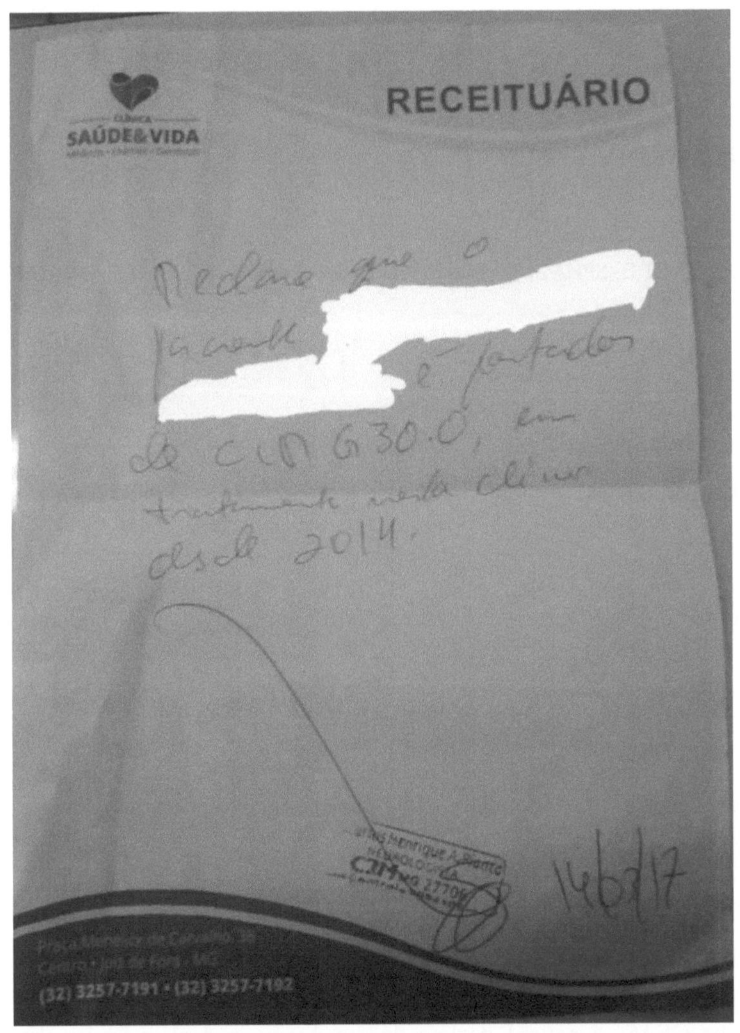

ANNEX: B SPEECH THERAPIST'S REPORT

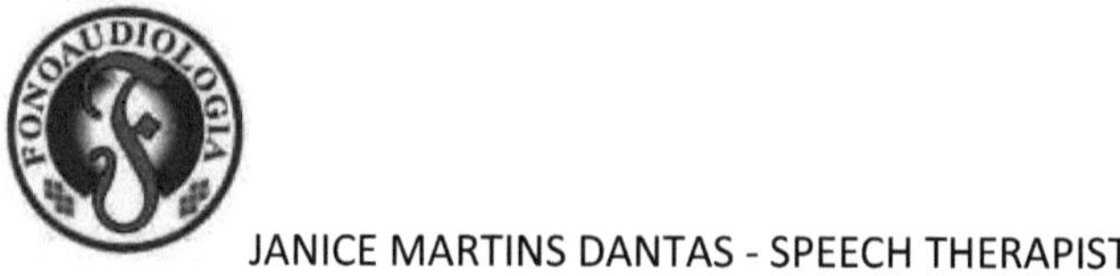

JANICE MARTINS DANTAS - SPEECH THERAPIST

CRF-4799- SPECIALIST IN DYSPHAGIA - EXPERT SPEECH THERAPIST SEPLAG-SPEECH

THERAPIST PJF

██████████████████ - (27/07/1935) HOME CARE PATIENT

Diagnosis: Alzheimer's disease, currently having difficulty swallowing (moderate oropharyngeal dysphagia).

At the initial assessment (2015), the patient showed a decrease in tongue and lip muscle strength, good laryngeal elevation and effective swallowing for oral feeding. At first, active and passive exercises were recommended to improve the strength and functionality of the OFAS, a natural decline due to ageing and also due to the progression of Alzheimer's disease. At the moment, feeding has only been adapted (more pasty consistencies, without large pieces or bran, liquids swallowed in small sips and slowly, position during and after feeding) and the use of a feeding tube is not indicated.

I returned for an assessment in February 2017, where the patient is already showing a significant progression of Alzheimer's disease, which is also directly interfering with his dysphasia, with refusal to eat, more frequent choking on all consistencies, The caregiver reports that at the moment she is having difficulty even giving the patient medication (sometimes he refuses, spits or locks his mouth), In this current situation, we are studying the possibility of introducing an alternative feeding route aiming at the adequate nutrition and hydration of the patient, as well as his greater comfort and safety in feeding.

Juiz de Fora ,2017

ANNEX: C PRESSURE ULCER IN THE COCCYGEAL REGION:

Start of treatment: End of treatment:

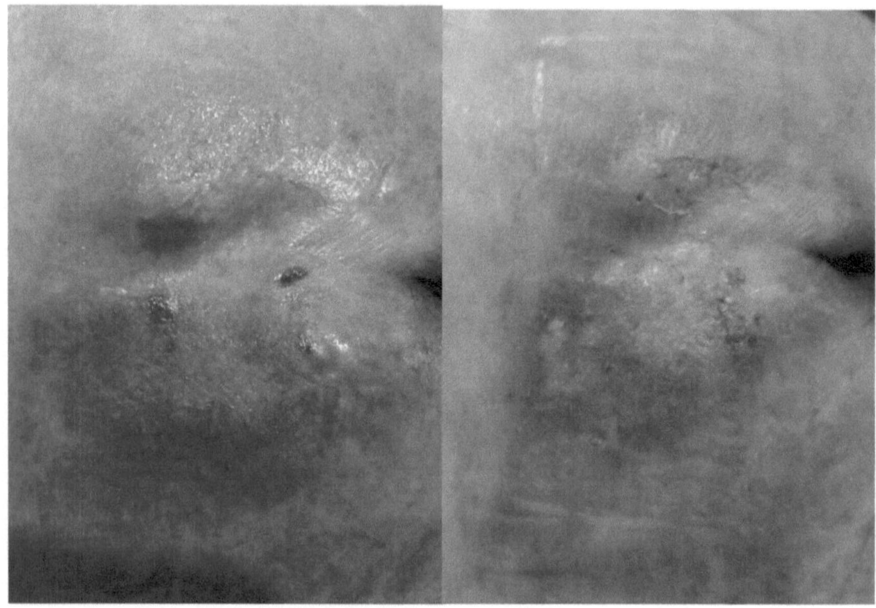

ANNEX: D PHOTOS OF THE PATIENT:

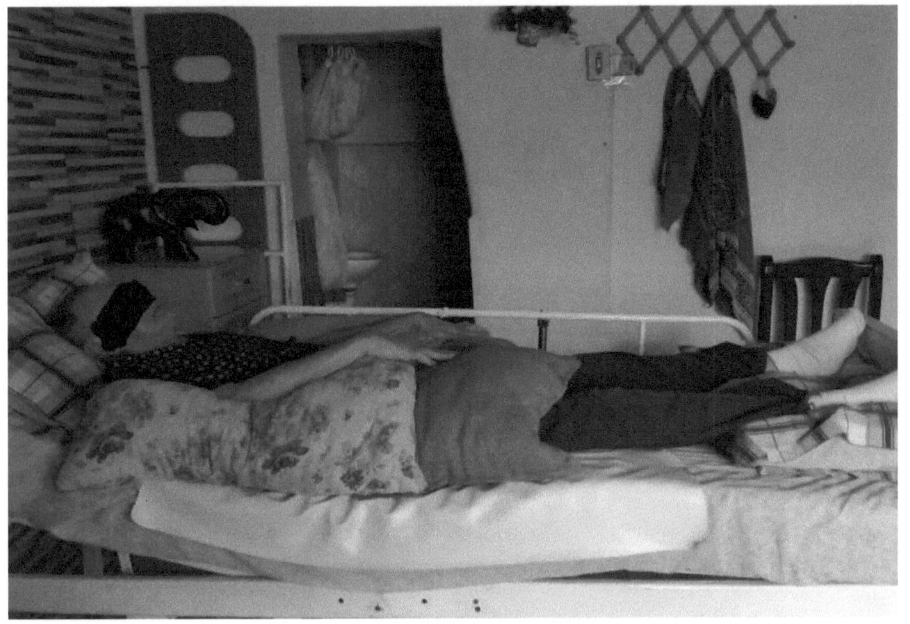

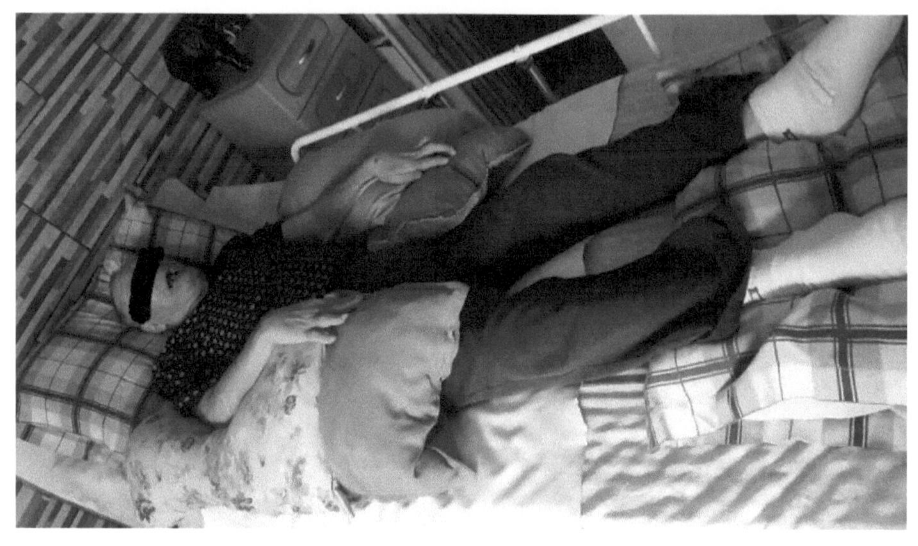

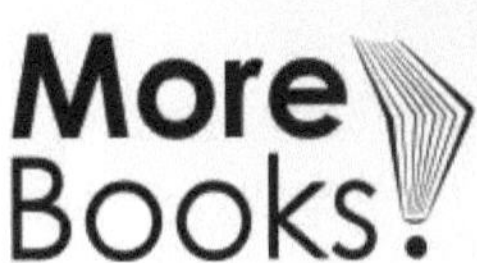

More
Books!

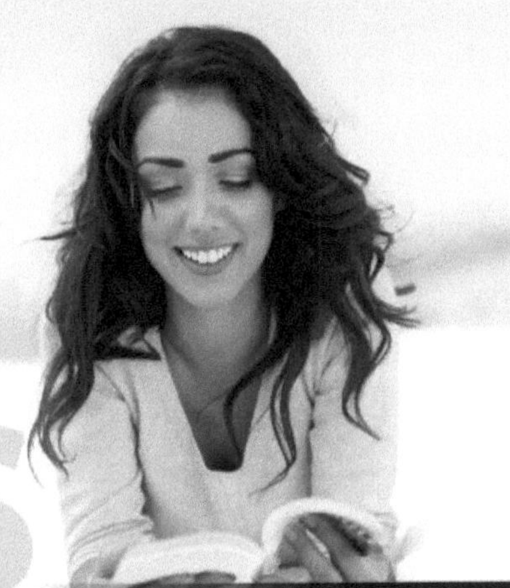

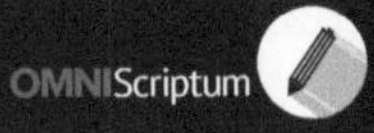

info@omniscriptum.com
www.omniscriptum.com
OMNIScriptum

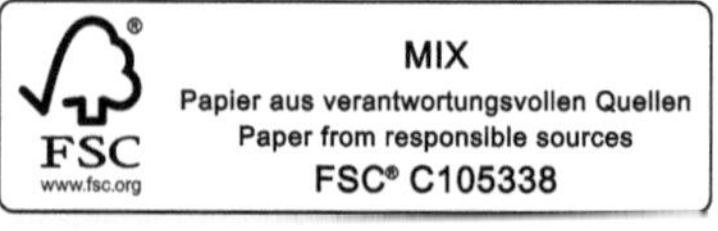

Printed by Books on Demand GmbH, Norderstedt / Germany